I0429052

Acne Cure

The Sure and Fast Way to Treat Your Acne Away

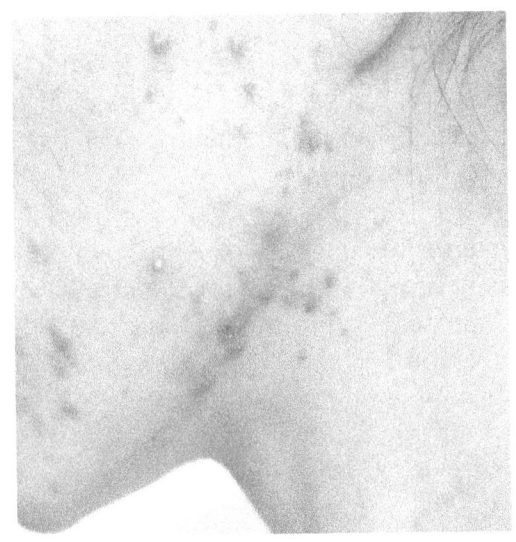

By
Fhilcar Faunillan

Copyright 2015 by Content Arcade Publishing - All rights reserved.

This document is geared towards providing exact and reliable information in regards to the topic and issue covered. The publication is sold with the idea that the publisher is not required to render accounting, officially permitted, or otherwise, qualified services. If advice is necessary, legal or professional, a practiced individual in the profession should be ordered.

- From a Declaration of Principles which was accepted and approved equally by a Committee of the American Bar Association and a Committee of Publishers and Associations.

In no way is it legal to reproduce, duplicate, or transmit any part of this document in either electronic means or in printed format. Recording of this publication is strictly prohibited and any storage of this document is not allowed unless with written permission from the publisher. All rights reserved.

The information provided herein is stated to be truthful and consistent, in that any liability, in terms of inattention or otherwise, by any usage or abuse of any policies, processes, or directions contained within is the solitary and utter responsibility of the recipient reader. Under no circumstances will any legal responsibility or blame be held against the publisher for any reparation, damages, or monetary loss due to the information herein, either directly or indirectly.

Respective authors own all copyrights not held by the publisher.

The information herein is offered for informational purposes solely, and is universal as so. The presentation of the information is without contract or any type of guarantee assurance.

The trademarks that are used are without any consent, and the publication of the trademark is without permission or backing by the trademark owner. All trademarks and brands within this book are for clarifying purposes only and are owned by the owners themselves, not affiliated with this document.

Table of Contents

INTRODUCTION

Everybody wants a smooth and pimple-free skin. It is not necessarily vanity, but having a smooth and fair skin is an indicator of health. The healthiness of your internal organs is reflected on the absence of physical blemishes on the outside. A healthy smooth skin also signifies youth and beauty.

Unfortunately for some, hideous pimples just appear on their skin, and it does not just end there. What is more problematic is that these pimples may leave scarring and discoloration. And even when already healed, pimples can still give you skin problems.

These pimples do not only give you physical setbacks but also lowers your self-esteem. Though most of the time acne only appears and wreaks havoc in the height of your teenage years, the scars

7

may still remain as you age, plaguing your skin and your confidence. Meeting people and former friends can also be harder because you will always have to be conscious of protruding bumps and pitted holes.

Acne victimizes any individual from any age group, but it is most common in teenagers due to their imbalanced hormones. But there are some unfortunate individuals who do not outgrow acne. It is a growing concern since a lot of people are experiencing devastating consequences because of it. Acne may be the most prevalent skin condition, but there are still misconceptions on how it works and its treatment.

In this book, you will learn about the beginnings of pimples, its prevention, cure and the useful habits necessary to keep your face free from acne. This will guide you on how to keep those zits away and have smooth fair skin.

Thank you for reading this book and enjoy!

Chapter 1 - How Do Pimples Form?

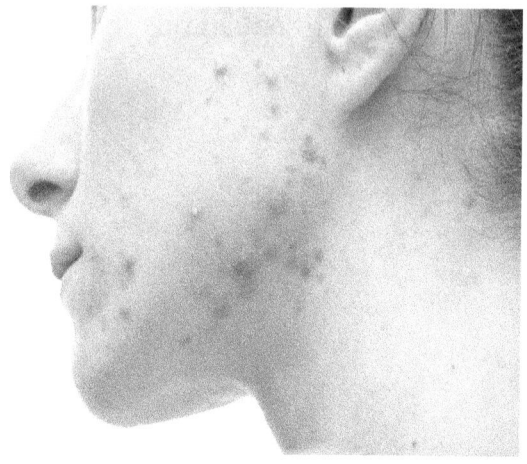

Pimples are small injuries and inflammations present in the skin. These are also known as comedones, spots and zits, and are most common in face, chest, shoulders, and back. Pimples occur in the pores or hair follicles, which are tiny openings in the skin. These pimples are formed in the sebaceous glands (oil glands) under the surface of the pores. When the sebaceous glands produce excess oil, it attracts bacteria and gets infected, clogged up by dirt, gets swollen, and then filled with pus.

It is natural for sebaceous glands to produce oil but when dirt and bacteria are combined with oil, it causes breakouts. There are also times that dead skin cells are left behind and get stuck with the oil causing blockage to the pore.

Your acne may be a telltale sign of your health. Break-outs on a specific part of the face reflect to a specific part of the body that is unhealthy or is compromised by irritants that has come in internally or externally.

Factors that can lead to acne:

1. Hormones.

There are many who suffer from recurring acne and cannot find the solution to that problem. Some people don't think that the cause of the problem can stem from the inside, but it can, and it's called hormones. Many women have not suffered from hormonal acne and thus, cannot recognize it. The hormone that is responsible for acne is androgen and high androgen levels are commonly linked with the growth of pimples.

People notice that women sometimes can tell upcoming menstrual period through the presence of pimples. This is because the hormonal imbalance during that period of the menstrual cycle causes the surge of pimples. About more than 60% of women experience this within 10 days before starting their menstrual period.

The location of the hormonal pimples is usually beneath the cheekbones and along the jaw line. Pimples along the nose and the forehead are more likely not related to the fluctuation of hormones. Pimples near the mouth area denote that there are problems around the reproductive system. Some people who are near their menstrual cycle have a pimple below their lower lip. Knowing this, treatment for hormonal acne is easier to do so.

What is hard about hormonal acne is that they tend to be large and cystic which can leave deep pitted scars. These pimples are sensitive to touch and you may feel a sensation of pain or pressure even without touching it. These pimples may sting when washing your face, and if you try to remove the pimple by popping, it will only result to scarring. Moreover, these pimples may not respond to topical creams and may appear dry and flaky.

There is also a condition called hypothyroidism in which the thyroid does not produce the necessary amount of hormones for the body. This condition could cause severe acne, as well.

Most people speak to their OB-GYNE for medication that could lessen the break-out. Doctors will most likely give you birth control pills that can mediate your hormonal imbalance.

2. Heredity

People with genetic predisposition to have acne are more likely to have one. If your family is suffering from acne, there is a huge chance to have one yourself. Studies have proven that acne is strongly genetic. If you have a first-degree relative with acne, it increases your risk to developing acne four times.

Even so, having the genes for acne does not necessarily mean that you will automatically get acne. However, if you are exposed to the other factors that contribute to acne, you are more likely to get it. Many experts emphasize the importance of heredity, since most often a family is also exposed to the same environmental factors (e.g. eating the same food and using the same products).

So how do both genes and hormones play in the role of acne? It all plays down to susceptibility. The androgen hormone has different effects on the skin of different people. If you are genetically predisposed to acne, androgen can be dangerous to your skin. As it is usually sebum production that is genetic and not the severity. Genetics also affect the body's inflammatory reaction to the bacteria, which may cause the pimples with bacteria to become more inflamed than normal.

3. Some Medicines

Acne is sometimes a result of the side effects of selected medicines. If your doctor puts you under medication like ion lithium or an anticonvulsant, acne is a possible side effect. Other drugs that could lead to acne or acne like conditions are corticosteroids, barbiturates, androgenic steroids, DHEA and other medications that contain bromides or iodides. The lithium is prescribed for bipolar patients while DHEA is an anti-aging hormone. Bromides and iodides are found in medications such as sedatives and cough medicines.

Majority of these skin eruptions are actually not really acne but are acne-like. These acne-like skin eruptions are seldom on the face and are more on the chest and the back. Acne can have different sizes and shape and types but the drug-related acne-like skin eruptions tend to look the same. It could happen to an individual with no history of acne.

Though majority of the side-effects of drugs are only acne-like, sometimes real acne is also caused by taking drugs.

Health professionals have yet to pinpoint the main cause of acne from medications, but currently the theory that the male hormone androgen contributes to the fluctuations in hormone levels still hold.

4. Cosmetic Products

Aside from cosmetic products clogging your pores and forming pimples, some ingredients may also actually irritate your skin. It is recommended that you consider the ingredients that you find irritating and avoid them in your products.

You should choose cosmetic products that are non-comedogenic, which means that they don't clog pores. However, many manufacturers will say their product is non-comedogenic so that they could sell them. Unsuspecting consumers may buy the products because of the promise that they can clear the blemishes, which actually contain chemicals that induce the growth of pimples.

Here are some of the ingredients that can cause acne:

- Lanolin- lanolin is a fatty substance that comes from the wool of sheep. While it is known to be an emollient (makes skin soft) with moisturizing properties, it can cause pore-clogging results, which result to break-outs.
- Fragrance- fragrances are irritants. Artificial fragrances can increase infection, skin sensitivity and photosensitivity.
- Mineral Oil- this is commonly used by a lot of people since it is a safer way of moisturizing and softening the skin, it is also used to remove make up. However, mineral oil is a thick substance that can also clog your pores.

- Dyes- dyes are known irritants, especially to sensitive skin. These dyes have comedogenic properties present that are derived from coal tar.

Here are things to remember so that you can avoid getting acne from using skin products:

- Avoid products that are creamy in texture or any products that appear in stick form. The creamy texture is caused by ingredients that are likely to cause acne. This makes your skin the perfect environment for those blemishes to grow. Dirt and bacteria are also more likely to stick to creamy substances.
- There are oils that are good for your skin. Pomegranate seed oil is a perfect example of oil that is nutritious for your skin and at the same time can prevent acne. You

may just find the oil greasy, and too much of it may interfere with your sebum.

- Avoid products that have irritating ingredients. Alcohol, menthol, peppermint, eucalyptus, lemon, camphor, lime and grapefruit are irritating to the skin. Irritation can cause sebum production at the base of the hair follicle and clog the pores. It can also redden your skin and inflame existing acne.

5. Pollution

As we all know, there are different kinds of pollution: air, water and land, and all of these can contribute to the formation of the dreaded acne. It's easy to be careful about getting in contact with water and land pollutants, but it's the air pollutants that are very hard to avoid since they can be present in the very air you breathe.

Everywhere you go, air pollutants will always be present.

Being in contact with pollutants is risking the development of acne. It might not be visible to the human eye, but there are tiny toxins in the air that can easily stick to your skin. It might get irritated and result to acne if the toxins and dirt present in the air is strong enough. That is why our skin breaks out more when the air is dirty.

Pollutants getting in contact with the skin are not the only probable cause of acne. When you inhale polluted air, your skin might still get affected. Toxins present in the inhaled air can get into your bloodstream. Blood is carried through capillaries in the skin, and when toxins make it to the capillary beds, the immune cells will try to take them out and the result is acne.

It is important to keep away from polluted areas as much as possible, but because pollutants are everywhere, it might be hard to do.

6. Diet and Exercise

Diet and exercise are one of the indirect factors in developing acne. Though there were some studies that have proven that diet has little to do with acne, but those researches are from forty years ago. Recent researches have linked the food with the development of acne.

For one, greasy food makes your sebaceous glands produce more oil than what is necessary. Being oily alone cannot lead to break-outs, but oil and dirt mixed up can clog pores resulting to acne.

Studies also show that those who consume low sugar and Low GI (Glycemic Index) food in their diet are less prone to acne. This is because sugary foods can trigger your sugar levels to shoot up and cause a sudden burst of the hormone insulin in the bloodstream, causing pimple breakout.

Here are some basic guides to eating in consideration to acne prevention:

- Eat more fruits and vegetables. These foods are very nutritious to the skin and are more likely to have healthy sugar levels. Identify the food that has high sugar content and avoid them. These foods are usually the processed ones such as junk foods, sodas, candies and canned goods. Eating fruits, vegetables and the occasional meat can steady your blood sugar levels and prevent inflammation at the same time. Eating properly not only rids your body of acne but also helps out your health as well. It will get rid of the toxins from the food that you eat out from your system. Remember, internal health reflects on the skin.

- Eat every two-three hours. Have small meals and eat them at little time intervals. When you eat less frequently but a lot, your body will release a surge of insulin. Eating small meals frequently steadies the insulin levels in your system.

- Be careful of eating dairy products such as cheese and milk. Though there are yet no substantial link between acne and dairy, there is anecdotal evidence that there is a connection. Some patients report to their doctor that their acne cleared up after stopping dairy. To exactly test this, you can skip dairy but find an alternative source of calcium.

- If you are someone with acne, you should consider a healthy diet.

Now, if you think about it, you should avoid fast food. These foods have little nutrition in them and instead have high fats and sugar content.

When it comes to exercise, a healthy life is definitely not complete without it. Though the sweat from exercise is not good for individuals with acne, the health benefit outweighs it. Sweating is a form of removing the toxins from the body, and these toxins may be the reason for your break-outs. When you exercise, the toxins exit the body through your pores. So keep in mind to wash yourself and use clean clothes after sweating, or the toxins may cling to your skin if you do not.

Chapter 2 - What are the Kinds of Pimples?

TYPES OF ACNE PIMPLES

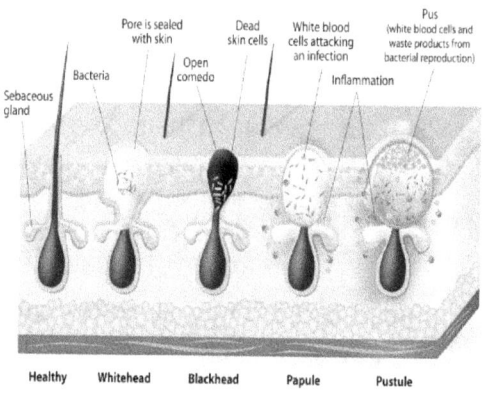

There are different kinds of pimples. These pimples have varying characteristics that respond to different treatment. Some, like blackheads and whiteheads, are simple to cure, while others such as cystic pimples are painful and difficult to treat. Blackheads and whiteheads are also less horrendous to see than the large cystic pimples.

Blackheads

Oil, dead skin cells and bacteria clog up pores and cause small bumps called blackheads. Blocked pores that stay open are called blackheads. The dark color at the tip is not due to the bacteria but to the oil reacting to air. This type of acne can easily be medicated on over-the-counter drugs.

Whiteheads

Similar to blackheads, whiteheads are clogged pores that have a layer of dead skin cells at the opening. Many medications against blackheads are also effective against whiteheads.

Papules

Papules are inflamed pimples that cause small, red bumps on the skin. This type of pimple is sensitive to touch and may worsen when touched or picked. When irritated, this type of pimple may cause scarring on the skin. Significant number of papules may indicate that the individual has a moderate to severe acne.

Pustules

Pustules are a lot worse than papules. They have a white head and red inflamed ring around them. They can also look like inflamed pimples with yellow or white pus underneath the inflammation. Never pick or irritate the pustules since it will cause severe scarring and discoloration on the affected area.

Nodules

Nodules are inflamed bumps that are firm to the touch unlike pustules. This type of pimple develops deep within the skin and is painful. These pimples should not be treated on your own. A dermatologist can be asked to treat these nodules. A doctor's prescription drugs may be powerful enough to get rid of them.

Cysts

Cysts are pus-filled lesions that look similar to boils. Like to nodules, cysts are painful and only dermatologists should be able to treat them correctly. When treated alone, it may get infected and worsen, plus this type of pimple can also lead to deep scarring on the skin. Individuals with cystic pimples are considered to have severe acne. This is also the worst type of acne to have.

Categories

Categories are made to assess the severity of the acne and to appropriate the treatment needed.

Mild Acne

Acne is considered mild when there are less than 20 whiteheads or blackheads and fewer than 15 inflamed bumps or less than 30 lesions. Mild acne can be treated using over the counter medicines or you can consult a health professional. The healing time of mild acne may vary from person to person and the severity of the condition. Expect your mild acne to heal at an average of two months of medication.

Moderate Acne

Acne is considered moderate when there are 20 to 100 whiteheads or blackheads, 15 to 50 total bumps or 30 to 125 total lesions. It is not advised to self-medicate when you have moderate to severe acne. See a skincare doctor and ask for prescription drugs for this acne category. Significant results may take longer and appear worse before getting better. Be patient.

Severe Nodule/Cystic Acne

Individuals with this acne have several nodules and cystic pimples. The pimples may turn red and purple and may result in deep scarring. Immediate treatment by skincare professionals prevents the scarring. Doctors may inject on pimples to lessen the inflammation and pain. Treatment may involve prescription drugs and medical procedures.

Chapter 3 - What Happens When You Do Not Treat Acne?

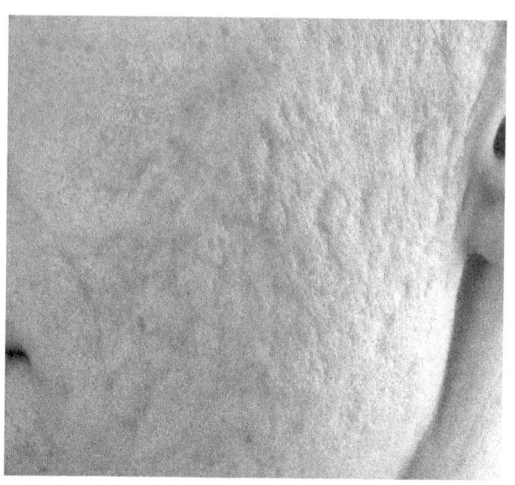

Acne Scars

Scarring is the worst consequence a pimple can give you. Though it is often misunderstood that these scars are permanent, there are still treatment procedures you can choose to eradicate specific kinds of scars if you want to. There are different kinds of scarring that may vary according to size, shape and color. Each type of acne scars is more

32

responsive to different kinds of treatment. It is most important to choose the right treatment that best matches your need depending on what type of acne scars you have. There are three main types of acne scars: raised acne scars, depressed acne scars and the discoloration scars.

Raised Acne Scars

Raised scars are also called keloid or hyper-trophic scars. These scars result from the building up of collagen fibers uncontrolled over a wound or skin disturbance such as a pimple. In simpler terms, there is an excess tissue on the pimple site that causes the scar to rise. Aside from being unsightly, these scars tend to be itchy.

Scars like these are more susceptible to treatments such as laser ablation and micro-dermabrasion. Raised acne scars can also be removed through cosmetic surgery. Unfortunately, this type of scars is less responsive to chemical treatments since scar tissue is more resistant to chemicals than healthy tissue.

Depressed Acne Scars

1. Ice pick Acne Scars

These kind of acne scars are the most unsightly and more difficult to remove. They are also not easy to cover with make-up. Ice pick scars are very deep scarring which makes normal resurfacing technique very difficult. Chemical peels, micro-dermabrasion and other common resurfacing methods have little impact on ice pick scars. Some laser treatments are the best options for ice-pick scars.

2. Rolling Acne Scars

Rolling acne scars are caused by being afflicted by inflammatory acne for a long time. These acne scars tend to be more pronounced as you age since the skin loses its fullness and elasticity the older you get. Rolling scars are rounded, sloping and less deep which makes them susceptible to simpler treatments such as chemical peels, micro-dermabrasion and other skin treatments.

3. Box Car Acne Scar

Box scars are acne scars with a more clearly defined and steeper edge. Because of these, smoothing and blending them into the surrounding skin is hard. Lasers are best matched in treating this type of scars.

Box cars are smaller than rolling scars and less deep than ice pick scars. By this, chemical peels, micro-dermabrasion, needling and other surgical treatment may help you fade the scars.

Discoloration and Pigmentation Scarring

Luckily for you, discoloration scars are the easiest to treat. This is because they are more on the outer part of the skin which is easier to slough off and be replaced.

1. Hyper-pigmentation

The trauma caused by the scarring of the skin tissue may not only produce excess growth of the tissue but also abnormal conditions in the skin. Hyper-pigmentation is a condition where elevated levels of the skin pigment melanin accumulate in the skin. When cells that produce melanin pigment (melanocytes) begin to proliferate at the injured area or near existing melanocytes, excessive amounts of melanin is produced. These may look like freckles but may be more severe.

Hyper-pigmentation can be addressed through prescription drugs such as hydroquinone which slows production of melanin, and topical retinoids which increase rate of skin turn-over. Hyper-pigmentation can also be treated with laser treatments such as KTP, pulsed dye lasers and intense pulse light (IPL) which specifically target melanin.

2.Hypo-pigmentation

While hyper-pigmentation is an excess in melanin, hypo-pigmentation occurs when melanocytes in the injured area are depleted and are unable to produce the needed amount of melanin. White or pinkish skin will appear on the injured part. Hypo-pigmentation is also more noticeable on darker skin. Unfortunately, there are no effective treatments for this condition.

3. Permanent Redness (Erythema)

Erythema happens when the small capillaries near the previously injured area of the skin becomes permanently dilated, or worse, damaged. This condition will show red colored skin patches. There are even times that individual capillaries are visible. It is common in acne patients especially those with lighter skin color.

Fortunately, there are both temporary and permanent treatments for erythema. Topical prescription medications to decrease vasodilation are available as temporary fix for the redness, and there are also lasers and light based-treatments such as argon and pulsed dye lasers as alternatives.

Chapter 4 - How to Treat Acne

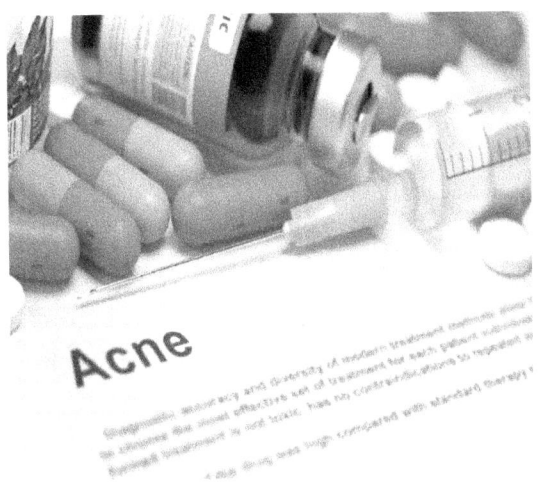

There are different ways to treat acne which range from home remedies to clinical help. You just have to seek the best way that suits you, since one treatment may be effective to others but not to you and vice versa. The costs of these treatments also depend on the severity of your acne.

Here are some medications used to treat acne (warning: consult a professional before taking any treatment):

Benzoyl Peroxide

This active ingredient can be found in many over the counter drugs. This is one of the easiest ways to get rid of acne. Benzoyl Peroxide prevents the spread of bacteria by killing them, unplugging oil ducts, and healing injured skin. Thus it's a very effective way to rid yourself of acne.

Directions:

1. Choose a product. It can be a facial lotion, gel or cream. Start with 5% mixture as to not irritate the skin. Make sure that your skin is clean when you apply the product.

2. After a week or so, increase the frequency of using the medication. You may opt to apply it in the morning and before going to bed.

3. If acne is not better after a month or two, increase the dosage into 10 %.

Retin A

Retin A is one of the most popular skin medications available. Apart from stopping acne, it also helps decrease spots, wrinkles and other blemishes. You can buy this product over the counter or with prescription. This is also a common whitening agent and used by many to achieve fairer skin.

Reminders:

1. Ask a skin professional to provide you the best kind of Retin A. Some products can cause dryness, peeling and redness. Make sure that you avoid them.

2. Use Retin A only at night. Retin A will make your skin sensitive to the rays of the sun. Make sure that you apply sunscreen in the morning to prevent sunburn.

3. Follow your doctor's instructions. It may take you as long as 2-3 months of Retin A use before seeing the result. In addition, pregnant women should avoid using Retin A since it is harmful to fetal

development. Your doctor may prescribe you with birth control pills, instead.

Antibiotics

Antibiotics are not available over-the-counter. It comes with a doctor's prescription only. Antibiotics can greatly help you improve acne especially those ones which are red and swollen. Antibiotics kill the bacteria, and at the same time prevent it from spreading. Taking antibiotics is often accompanied with other medication.

However, growing concern arises with the use of antibiotics. This is because it can actually strengthen the bacteria when not fully eradicated. Some people mistakenly think that just because the acne disappears, the bacteria aren't there. So make sure that you finish your prescription.

Reminders:

1. Drink plenty of water when taking antibiotics.

2. Make sure to follow your doctor's instructions.

3. Antibiotics can make your skin sensitive to the sun. Protect your skin by applying sunscreen.

Accutane

Accutane is often the last resort when treating acne. Like antibiotics, it is only available with a doctor's prescription. This drug is very powerful that it is only intended for people with severe acne. Some physicians will not even prescribe accutane.

Reminders:

1. Accutane has serious side effects, like affecting your blood cell count. To monitor your blood health, frequent blood testing is needed.

2. Physicians may also require females to have two forms of birth control before

prescribing Accutane. This is because it can severely damage fetal development in pregnant women.

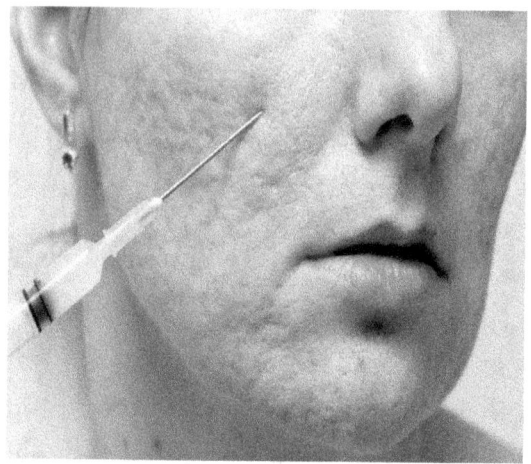

Steroid Injection

Steroid injection is used for painful lumps beneath the surface of the skin such as nodules and cysts. Though cysts and nodules can heal on their own, they are prone to infection and scarring, and these scars may take weeks before totally healing.

After the injection, the bumps will flatten and pain will lessen in just two to four days. This drug is super effective against cystic acne but may have some side effects.

These are the probable side effects of steroid injections:
- painful procedure (although doctors can apply anesthetic)
- thinning around the treated skin
- appearance of small blood vessels on the treated area
- skin tone appearing lighter than normal

Remember that steroid injections are only used to fix stubborn cystic acne. It is not advised to be used as a cure for widespread acne due to its side effects. Frequent doctor visits are also necessary to monitor the treated skin.

Acne Draining

This is similar to popping a pimple but should be done with skilled hands. The pimple (usually cystic acne) is lanced, incised with a sharp needle and drained to cure it. Draining is usually done when the cystic acne does not respond to topical and oral treatments. This procedure should never be done at home or without professional help, since improper draining of a cystic acne may cause infection and deep scarring.

Chapter 5 - Treatments Available forAcne Scarring

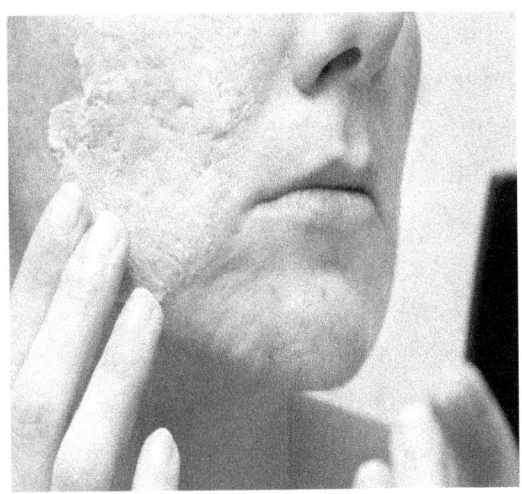

There are different treatments available for acne scarring. You just have to choose what you think is best for what you have.

Cortisone Creams

These creams are topical ointments that are used for red and swollen scars. Cortisone is absorbed by the skin and calms the inflammation. Cortisone creams are usually used for inflamed joints in arthritis but can also be used for other skin conditions such as rashes and eczema. It is available in over the counter drugs and can be used per the manufacturer's instructions. Cortisone creams can also be used for active acne, though it is best effective against inflamed and cystic acne.

Ask a health professional for advice before using cortisone creams to prevent complications. It is not advised to be used by pregnant women and other individuals who are taking other medications since some medications may react to cortisone. If the red, inflamed skin does not get better in seven days, go see a doctor.

Directions:

1. Clean your face thoroughly and exfoliate to remove dead skin cells. Choose mild exfoliant to prevent irritation and inflammation.

2. Dab the cortisone cream on the area needed. Apply twice daily. If acne

worsens, stop usage. Some skins do not go well with cortisone treatments.

Hydroquinone

Hydroquinone is one of the most popular ways of getting rid of discoloration. It is a skin lightener that is used in whitening creams to fade acne marks, and it is great for hyper-pigmentation. But through the years, hydroquinone has achieved many criticisms. This is because there are recent investigations that indicate that hydroquinone causes multiple side effects.

Though there are side effects, nothing is conclusive but it is advised that you use hydroquinone products with care. Consult your doctor before using hydroquinone products. If you are pregnant or planning to be, please do not use this product. It may harm your fetus. Further, do not use hydroquinone if you are under medication, since it may not go well with your medicine. For example, hydroquinone does not work well with Benzoyl Peroxide. If used together, it may cause the skin to burn and darken.

Directions:

1. Check first for allergic reactions. Some individuals are allergic to hydroquinone. Apply it on your arm to test your allergic reaction.

2. Wash your face and let it dry out. Apply the hydroquinone cream evenly on your face. Massage the affected area gently and wash your hands after. If you miss an application, you can apply it as soon as you can.

3. Do not use it on active acne since it can irritate the skin more.

4. Use it on the skin only. Rinse thoroughly when it comes contact with eyes and lips. If further irritation occurs, consult your doctor.

5. Lastly, this medication can increase your skin's sensitivity to the sun, so make

sure that you use sunscreen with a high SPF.

Hydroquinone may have side effects. Dryness, flaking and cracking of the skin may occur. It may cause your skin to redden and you will feel a mild burning sensation. Go see a doctor when you experience these and the following symptoms: severe allergic reactions, darkening of the skin, blistering, stinging and excessive irritation.

Micro-dermabrasion

Micro-dermabrasion, one of the most popular procedures, uses tiny crystals to slough off the layer of the skin. It is not only for getting rid of acne scars but also for keeping wrinkles, age spots and dullness away. Micro-dermabrasion may show a great improvement on the first session but you need to undergo a few more to definitely get rid of acne scars.

Microdermabrasion is also great for those suffering from active acne since the procedure can unclog the pores. Those individuals with deeper acne scars may need further sessions and laser procedure to smooth the skin.

Individuals using microdermabrasion gave positive feedbacks. Their skin was reported to be smoother and the spots are lighter. It may give off a pink finish but the skin will recover immediately after 24 hours.

Intense Pulsed Light (LPL)

Intense Pulse Light (IPL), also called photofacial, is a great procedure for light to moderate types of acne scarring. During a session of photofacial, a short intense light is emitted from an applicator onto the skin. The intense light with a specific wavelength emitted will destroy the pigmented skin cells. After few sessions with Intense Pulsed Light, brown and red marks in your skin will disappear. IPL is also great for active acne. With a specified wavelength, the intense light will kill off the bacteria in the skin and treat the inflamed skin. The light will mostly target bacterial growth and inflamed sebaceous glands.

When you visit a clinic for a photofacial, your face will be cleansed thoroughly by a skin care professional. Gel will be applied on the face and the actual procedure will begin. It will only take up to 15 to 25 minutes. You will feel only slight and brief prickling as your skin adjusts to absorb the light. Another layer of gel will be applied on your skin to ease out your discomfort.

Reminders:

1. IPL can be used by anyone but those with dark skins. Dark skinned individuals may experience hyper-pigmentation after a session with IPL.

2. Those who are also under medication and recently been using Accutane should not undergo IPL.

3. Those who wish to be pregnant, actually pregnant and women who are photosensitive should first consult their doctor before undergoing the procedure.

4. These treatments have no downtime and you will only experience mild redness which can be covered by make-up. The best results will be achieved after three to five sessions of IPL.

5. IPL is often accompanied with other acne clearing medications to get the best results.

Chemical peels

Chemical peels are popular procedures done for skin improvement. They are also great for fading sunspots, red marks and hyper-pigmentation. The chemical solution is applied onto the skin, making it blister and peel off. The layers of dead cells are then sloughed off, making your skin smooth and radiant.

Before heading out to try chemical peels, make sure to consult your doctor first. You must know how deep the peeling should be or if you need other medications along the way.

As a standard procedure in any facial session, your face will be cleansed. The skin professional will then apply a chemical solution or a few other substances to your skin. The chemical solutions used can be one of the following: carbolic acid, glycolic acid, lactic acid, salicylic acid, and trichloroacetic acid. This solution will create controlled wound or blisters to let new skin set in.

During the chemical peel, individuals will feel a burning sensation for about ten minutes before feeling the stinging on the skin. Putting on cold compress on the areas may relieve the stinging sensation. For deeper and stronger peels, some may need pain medication.

Results may vary depending on the skin that you have and the type of chemicals applied on it. Some may experience effects similar to sunburns. There will also be redness on the skin, followed by scaling and eventually to peeling. This will last for seven days. Mild peels are repeated at one to four week intervals before achieving the desired result.

Medium depth and deep peels may result in swelling, blisters, cracking and peeling in a period of seven to fourteen days. Medium peels, if necessary, will be repeated at 6 months to 12 months interval. After treatment, you may need bandages on your skin.

The downside of this treatment is the pain and the downtime. You may also need to stay away from the sun for few months since the new skin will be so sensitive to its harsh rays.

Skin Needling

Skin needling is an old-fashioned procedure of resurfacing skin that uses multiple thin needles in a roller, piercing through the first layers of the skin. The roller needles vary in length, from .25 millimeters to 2.5 millimeters depending on the purpose. The longer the needles the deeper its reach on the acne scars.

Skin needling works by having each needle pierce the skin, stimulating collagen production. Collagen production helps in healing scars, wrinkles and skin damage. This may sound terrifying and invasive but it is fairly effective and safe.

During a needling session, skin professionals will clean your face and apply a mild anesthesia. They will begin the needling afterwards. The needles may sting but the pain is tolerable due to the anesthesia. There might be blood present, but it is only natural. After the procedure, your face might be red from the prickling, but it will heal after a few days. It may take a few weeks before needling again, and that depends on the length of the needles used on you. The longer the needles, the longer the time is for skin healing.

Skin needling is mostly done for moderate and severe acne scars. Researchers have proven that acne scarring is visibly reduced after sessions of skin needling. Though it can be done at home, skin specialists advise not to do so, since an inexperienced hand may cause scarring and skin infection. Doing it by yourself may worsen your condition.

Skin needling is also great for those with wrinkles, fine lines and other age related skin problems. But though it may be a miracle worker for aging symptoms, it is not great for treating active acne. The bacteria present in pierced pimples may only transfer to other healthy parts, which may cause severe acne break-out and infection.

Pulsed Dye Laser (PDL)

Pulsed Dye Laser is good for active acne, erythema and hyper-pigmentation. Several clinical studies have proven that PDL is the best for hard-to-remove erythema. Basically, it is a laser therapy treatment that uses organic dye mixed in solvent as the laser medium. The laser produces pulses of visible light at a wavelength of 585 or 595 nm with pulse durations on the order of .45-.40 ms.

The procedure of Pulsed Dye Laser is centered on the principle of thermolysis.

When the pulsed dye hits the skin cells, it is thereby reflected, transmitted and/or absorbed. The absorbed energy from the laser is then responsible for the killing of the diseased skin cells.

The process of having a pulsed dye laser procedure starts off by necessary cleansing and prepping. Afterwards, clinicians use laser-emitting hand tools against the skin. Several patients described the procedure as similar to the snapping of a rubber band against the skin. Anesthesia may be applied to the skin but it's not essentially necessary to the procedure. An ice pack may be applied on the skin for a soothing effect, instead.

Avoidance of using abrasive skin care products is advised to prevent irritation. Sun exposure should also be avoided since the skin can become sensitive to the sun. Exposure to the sun may cause postinflammatory pigmentation on the skin. Also, avoid any contact to the treated area until the skin is fully healed.

The most common side effect of the Pulsed Dye Laser is the pain during and after the procedure as well as the redness and slight inflammation. Blistering could also occur when the skin is exposed to the sun, but it can eventually be healed. Sometimes, bacterial infection occurs as well, that is why antibiotics are prescribed to the patients to prevent wound infection.

Chapter 6 - The Skincare Regimen to Prevent Acne

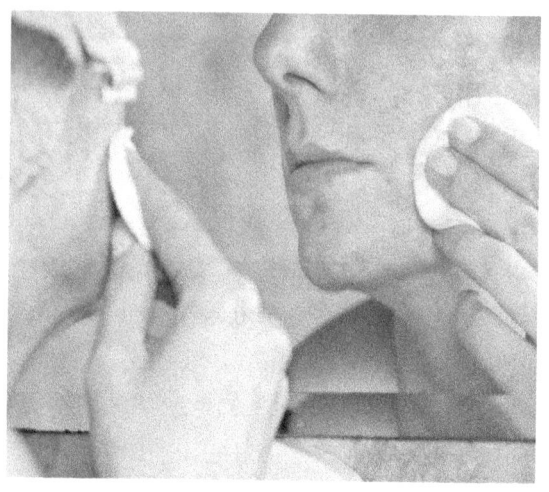

As you age, your skin needs more care to keep it healthy and beautiful. It does not only keep those red points off your face but also minimizes the appearance of signs of aging such as age spots, lines and wrinkles.

Now, you have to remember that even the skincare regimen and the products you use can result to break-outs. For example, pimples can be caused by products like your creams, astringents, and even your perfumes and your hair products. Some fragrance can cause your skin to go on a rampage, and some hair products can also give you acne especially on the parts where your hair touches the skin.

It's better to avoid creams and opt for gel or powder counterparts, instead. This is because creams contain ingredients that can clog pores, while gels are better since they have soothing properties for the skin.

What you need to know is that during the day, it is important to cleanse, treat, moisturize and protect your skin. You may want to leave the healing and nourishing products during the night for better absorption. The traditional nightly routine would be Cleanse-Tone-Moisturize, but another way of skin care has emerged which involves cleansing, toning, revitalizing and moisturizing. It is a more in depth routine that encourages better health of the skin cells.

Skin care routine varies for every individual. You have to assess your needs to know how to address them. Some people have very elaborate beauty regimens, using different types of products ranging from five to ten kinds, while some prefer simpler routines.

Below, you can find a guide for a basic skin care routine to prevent acne.

Cleansing

Keeping your skin clean is keeping your face without blemish. To do this, a light cleanse should be done in the morning when you wake up to keep your skin fresh, hydrated and clean. You may think that your skin is clean because you washed the night before. However, when you are sleeping, your skin sweats, sheds off dead skin cells, and contracts dust and dirt. That is why a light cleanse is vital in the morning. But be mindful to clean gently since harshly cleansing your face in the morning will strip the skin off of its natural oil, which leaves the skin unprotected from the sun and dirt.

Night cleansing is the most important part of any skincare regimen. During the day, dirt, dust, bacteria, oil and other substances are accumulated on the skin. That is why it is vital to thoroughly wash off these substances. Keeping your face clean allows your skin to breath away from make-up, sweat and pollution.

Cleansing during the night also preps the skin for the application of your toner, moisturizer and serum. Having a clean face ensures that the products you put on it are properly absorbed.

When using a cleanser, remember that when it leaves oil in your face, it is not doing its job. If it makes your face feel too tight, it is too harsh for your skin. When using a facial wash, make sure to rinse the residue off your skin properly. This is because facial washes tend to stick to the skin when not washed off totally.

There are several cleansers that are available in the market, in the form of cleansing oils, facial foams, facial washes and others. You just have to choose what is not irritating to your skin and what you are comfortable to use.

Toners

Toners are liquid substances that are designed to further cleanse the skin and shrink the size of the pores. It is like prepping the skin for the serum and moisturizers. Toners can be applied through one of these three ways: using cotton and dabbing it on the skin, spraying it on your face, or putting on facial masks which have toners as one of the ingredients.

There are three types of toners and these are:

Fresheners. These toners are the mildest and contain water, a humectant such as glycerine, and a little alcohol of about 0-10% in concentration. Humectants help the skin retain more fluids by preventing the moisture from evaporating. A popular example of a freshener is rosewater. They are the gentlest and can be used by any skin types. It may give off a very slight stinging to sensitive skin.

Skin Tonics. These toners are stronger than fresheners. They contain water, a humectant and up to 20% alcohol. Orange flower water is an example of a skin tonic. This toner is ideal for normal, combination and oily skin types.

Astringents. These are the strongest of the toners, and they contain water, a humectant, alcohol about 20-60% in concentration, and antiseptic ingredients. This toner is recommended for people with severe oily skin since these toners can dry your skin.

Using toners is not as popular as using moisturizers, but this is still important in any skincare regimen. Here are the reasons why you should use a toner:

- It shrinks the pores in your skin.
- It gives your skin its natural PH balance.
- It adds another layer of protection.
- Most toners have moisturizing properties.
- It revitalizes the skin.
- Some toners containing glycolic and AHA keep off ingrown hair.

Moisturizing

Moisturizers are what hydrates your skin. Skincare professionals recommend applying them daily to avoid wrinkles and skin problems. There are several products in the market that promises a smoother, more beautiful skin which may leave you confused. But all professionals agree that drying up your skin is not the cure for acne. Below are the tips on how to choose your moisturizers.

- The first thing to consider is your skin type. If you have a very dry skin, you should opt for a light cream. If you have oily skin, you should use a lotion.
- Moisturize after you put your acne treatment. The period after cleansing is when the skin is most absorbent to products. Apply treatment to your skin and let it rest before applying your moisturizer.

- Make sure that the moisturizer that you choose does not have oil in it. If you have oily skin, do not over moisturize, since it may only overwhelm your skin and cause break-outs.
- You should choose a moisturizer that prevents the development of acne. You should look for those with salicylic acid or benzoyl peroxide when choosing a moisturizer.
- Remember that natural products are not necessarily better when moisturizing with acne. Some natural products are irritants to the skin.

Serums

Serums are most likely to be confused with moisturizers. Serums are nourishing liquid to moisturize and revitalize the skin. A lot of people are intimidated with its hefty price tag and little bottles. Some people ignore serums because they think that it is not important for the skin. If you are young and have a very nice skin texture, you may not need it for the moment. But as you age, your skin needs nutrients to look beautiful and smooth.

When used regularly, serums improve the overall wellness of the skin. They prevent wrinkles, spots, blemishes and even protect your skin from free radicals. Serums are also moisturizers that are filled with nutrients. It is not necessary to moisturize after putting in serums, since they are already concentrates of nutritional benefits for the skin.

The downside of using serums is that they are expensive compared to other skincare products. There is a tendency of higher quality ingredients to be used in expensive serums compared to cheaper alternatives. There are different kinds of serums for different needs. You must choose what you think suits your needs best.

There are three things you should look for in a serum:

- **Hydrators**. These are the ingredients that moisturize your skin. It protects your skin by replenishing your skin lipids, improving moisture retention and shielding the skin from the hazards of the environment. Examples of hydrators include ceramides, amino acids and essential fatty acids.
- **Antioxidants**. These are the ingredients that fight against the sun and free radicals. They are responsible for prevention and fading of sun spots, wrinkles and acne marks. Examples of antioxidants would be pomegranate seed oil, Vitamin C and grape seed extract.

- **Anti-inflammatory**. These ingredients neutralize the inflammation, redness and prevent further cellular damage. This is important for acne-prone skin because this ingredient helps reduce the presence of acne. Examples of anti-inflammatory ingredients would be zinc, arnica, aloe vera and goldenseal.

You can apply serum night and day. But if you are applying retinoids during the evening, avoid using the serum. This may lead to irritation of the skin. If you have dry skin and think that the serum is not enough to moisturize it, you can opt to add moisturizer on top of the serum. Make sure that the serum penetrates the skin and give it time before applying the moisturizer. As a general rule of every product, do not overuse the serum. Use only as instructed in their labels.

Chapter 7 - Habits that Lead to Acne

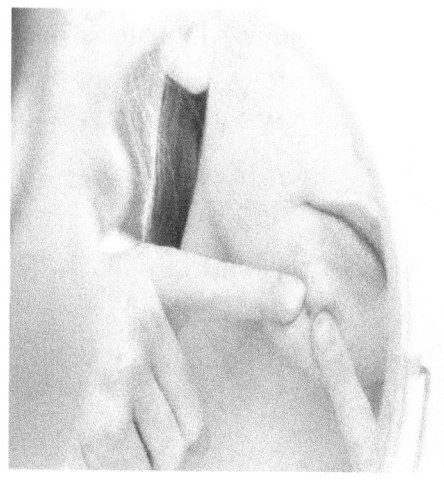

There are a lot of things we do to our skin that makes it susceptible to pimples and even worsens it. Here are a few of them:

1. Leaving your face dirty

Keeping your face clean is the number 1 rule in skincare and cleansing your face is the most important part of any skin care regimen. If you keep your face clean, it stops the bacteria from spreading and rids it of the excess oil which is a known contributor in acne breakouts.

There are many ways and several products to choose from to clean your face. Using soap is a popular method, but they are too harsh for your facial skin. However, there are also some soap that may be mild enough to clean your face, such as Dove and Cetaphil. There are also facial washes and cleansing oils available for you to use. You can choose what best suits your skin.

It is recommended to use cleansers that are made especially for acne-prone skin. There are cleansers that have salicylic acid or benzoyl peroxide, which helps lessen the aggravation of acne.

The best time to wash is during the night before you sleep and in the morning after you wake up. It is best not to wash more than twice since it can cause imbalance in the skin, which can aggravate it, and cause to have more pimples. Over cleaning strips the skin's natural oils that serves as barrier against bacteria.

What you use during cleansing must be gentle and effective. You are discouraged to use facial scrubs and wash cloths. Acne prone skin is sensitive to these and may only worsen acne. The harsh scrubbing might rupture the inflamed pimples, causing them to scar. It is best to use your hands in gently washing your face in a circular motion with a facial wash.

2. Getting the wrong products for your skin

Facial products have different impacts on different skin, so it is up to you to find what suits your skin best. If you have sensitive skin, choose mild products, and if you have normal skin, you might be able to take on stronger ones. Comedogenic products are those that can cause your skin to develop pimples since it can clog pores. You have to avoid these products by choosing those that says they're non-comedogenic. Also, remember that pimples are really sensitive to anything and harshly cleansing them will only worsen your condition. So, make sure that you cleanse gently.

Keep your skin clean all day. Your face should avoid contact with things that have rich bacterial growth. A few good examples would be your phone and your hands. You cannot avoid having contact with these items so you should make sure that they are clean before touching your face.

3. Skipping your daily regimen

Always be religious in following your daily regimen. If you skip a single anti-acne medication, it may lower your chances for treatment. Do not forget to remove your make-up daily since a miss can cause a break-out. This is why it is important to follow your routine without fail to avoid doing something that you will regret deeply. A hardworking individual may reap the benefits of a healthy glowing skin.

4. Handling your skin

Improper handling of your skin can lead to an acne breakout. Many things can come in contact with your skin that can be unwitting carriers of bacteria and germs. Here are a few things that you should be mindful of when handling your skin:

- Your hands can be filled with dirt and germs which can clog your pores. Never touch your face with your hand or anything dirty such as your phone.
- Most people forget to wash their cosmetic materials such as brushes. Dirt and dust accumulated can contribute to your acne. That is why it is

important to clean your brushes regularly. There are products that are made solely for cleaning make-up materials that will not ruin their quality. Sponges should always be replaced once in a while. Dried make-up and accumulated dirt may stick within the sponges.

- Your pillow cases should be changed every week if you have acne. Remember that sweat and dirt can also accumulate not only in your face but also in your hair, and products from your hair might stick onto your pillowcases.

5. Sweating without washing afterwards

Sweat is filled with bacteria and attracts more of them. It is important to wash your skin when you sweat. You should avoid using sweaty clothes and things as sweat may also stick on your accessories.

Keep in mind to clean your accessories regularly, too.

6. Eating unhealthy foods.

According to research, what you eat does not directly cause acne, but the oil in them. When you eat greasy foods, there is a higher chance of sebum production which increases the probability of having break-outs. Some people have break-outs due to the consumption of dairy products. Dairy products may cause hormonal imbalance in some and produce unwanted zits.

Skin can be taken care of from the inside and the outside. So choose healthy food and stay away from the greasy ones. More importantly, avoid fast food. Foods that are rich in antioxidants can help you heal your skin lesions easily. You can find these antioxidants in pomegranates, grapes, cranberries and other berries.

7. Popping your Zits

Never ever pop your zits. You might be itching to get rid of that big red pimple, but don't pop it. It may be effective at times but mostly it only worsens your skin condition.

When you pop your pimples, there is a tendency that you can push the pus and bacteria deeper with your hand, causing a more severe infection. Your nails and hands may also infect the pimples more. Popping your zits may also damage your skin cells and cause severe acne scars.

8. Contact with Pollutants

Pollutants are major contributors to acne. Stay away from polluted areas that could not only cause pimples but also other diseases. Keep away from belching cars and smoking individuals as much as possible. These pollutants lower the quality of your skin and worsen the inflammation of your pimples.

9. Self-Medicating

Self-medication is fine if you only have mild pimples. But it may become worse if you do it wrong.

When self-medicating, you cannot be sure of the possible reactions and side effects. Some medications may also be incompatible with your health and skin type. There are several things to consider when medicating, and this includes possible allergic reactions, your schedule, overall health and others.

The best thing to do is to consult your doctor especially if you have moderate to severe acne, since skin professionals know the best treatment for your acne. What you need to do is to follow it religiously.

Chapter 8 - Make-Up Use

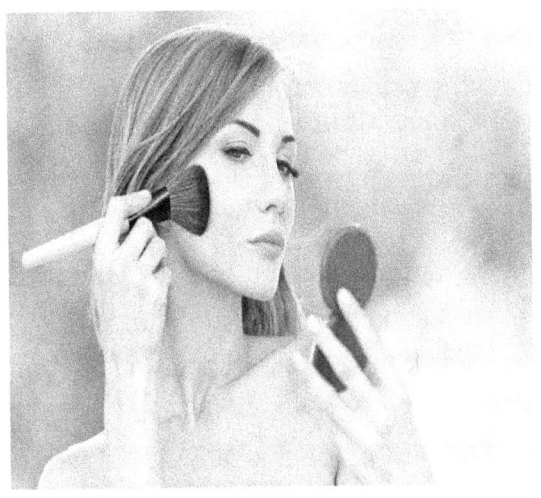

Product use was briefly discussed in previous chapters. In this chapter, you will find a guide in choosing the basic products for your sensitive skin is thoroughly explained. These products may include sunscreens, foundations, BB creams, CC creams, lipstick and other make-up products that people usually use.

Sunscreen

Sunscreen is the most important product when applying make-up, because sunscreen protects the skin from the harmful rays of the sun. It is important to use sunscreen religiously and correctly.

When you are plagued with pimples, it is best to keep away from the sun. Athough the sun kills off the bacteria on your pimples, it causes the sebum (oil) production to increase and this can worsen your acne condition. There are products that already contain sunscreen so it will not be difficult to include in your make-up application.

However, there are ingredients in these products that can cause your acne to worsen. These ingredients are the following:

- Zinc oxide
- Titanium dioxide

- Avobenzone (also labeled as Parsol 1789 or by its chemical name benzyl methoxydibenzoylmethane)
- Tinosorb (labeled by some manufacturers by its chemical name bisethylhexyloxyphenol methoxyphenyl triazine)
- Mexoryl (also known as ecamsule and by its chemical name terephthalyllidene dicamphor sulfonic acid)

If you see these ingredients in your sunscreen, might as well choose another product. Though these ingredients do not necessarily cause pimples and may have no effects on your skin, results still may vary from person to person.

Foundations

Foundations are staple make-up products that are used to cover up break-outs. Although this product is known for its great coverage, some may find foundation aggravating to their acne. It is always a question what foundations to use when you have a sensitive skin.

Fortunately, there are brands that develop foundation for individuals with acne, but most of them only supply coverage but not healing. Also, creamy foundation can cause clogging of the pores. Added to that, girls tend to wear more make-up to cover the blemishes, which can give your skin a nightmare.

Covering up is understandable, that is why it is recommended to use foundations that are not oil-based, hypo-allergenic and non-comedogenic. It is always best to use only a light layer of foundation. If you have oily skin, skip the creams and opt for gels and powder to cover-up, but if you are someone with dry skin, you should avoid cream and powder. A foundation for acne-prone skin should not contain ingredients that can make the skin break out, such as mint, menthol, lavender, lemon oil, linalool, or cinnamon.

BB Cream

BB creams were first used by Germans for healing the skin after surgery. Years later, the South Koreans found cosmetic use for it and it is now one of the hottest beauty products in the world. Though Asian in origin, several western companies has now produced their own version of BB cream. The "BB" in the product's name stands for Blemish Balm, which is intended for skin blemishes such as acne and acne scars.

The rave about BB cream is caused by its diverse functions. It can be used as coverage, a concealer, a serum, a sunscreen and an anti-acne product. With BB Cream, there is less hassle in applying make-up as it has become a single make-up product with a lot of uses.

If you are considering to buy BB creams, it is recommended to choose a brand from East Asia. Usually, products labeled BB cream in the Western World are just tinted moisturizers. BB creams from Asia tend to have more nutrients than the Western brands. But still, these brands should not be generalized, as there are some Western brands that have the same quality with that of their Asian counterparts. Read the labels and choose the product that offers the most benefit and falls within your budget.

Finally, although using BB cream is generally safer than any other make-up, some people are highly sensitive to it so it is best to be cautious in using this product.

Concealers

Concealers are for covering blemishes such as sunspots, acne scars and even eye bags. There are tones available for different skin color. If you are light-skinned, yellow concealers work best for your skin, while Asian skin works best with brown concealers. And if you have dark skin, you can use brown or no concealer at all. Choice color matters when applying concealer since if you get it wrong, you may end up with discoloration.

Powder

Powders are used to set your make-up and avoid oiliness. Using powder can cover your wrinkles, lines and blemishes. However, using excess powder may only end up with clogged pores.

Lipstick

Lips are pimple-free but lipstick can still do harm to your skin. Ingredients in lipsticks are capable of clogging pores and thus, can still to cause a break-out. The glossier the lipstick the more dangerous it is to acne-prone skin.

Make-up Removers

Make-up removers are great for easily removing make-up. The best make-up removers are fragrance free so as to not irritate the skin. Because some make-ups are hard to remove and require vigorous rubbing to come off, make-up removers can help you to gently remove your make-up without irritating the skin and causing more pimples.

Eye make-up

Usually, there are no pimples around the eye area. The problem is that the make-up will smudge over the other parts of your skin. So, it is best that you use them only in modicum amounts and that you avoid sweating to keep make-up from smudging.

Conclusion

Thank you for reading this book till the end. Its main purpose is to inform you of everything about acne. I hope that you got what you sought in this thorough discussion about acne. Now that you have the knowledge of how acne works and its prevention and cure, you are now equipped to fight against it.

As the saying goes, "An ounce of prevention is better than a pound of cure". If you have not yet experienced acne, then you're very lucky. You now have time to take care of your skin more to prevent acne and its devastating effects to take hold. But if you are currently suffering from acne, then you can now start to do your best to cure them.

I hope this book will help you to be healthy, beautiful, young, and acne free.

Live your life to the fullest. I wish you the best of luck and good health!

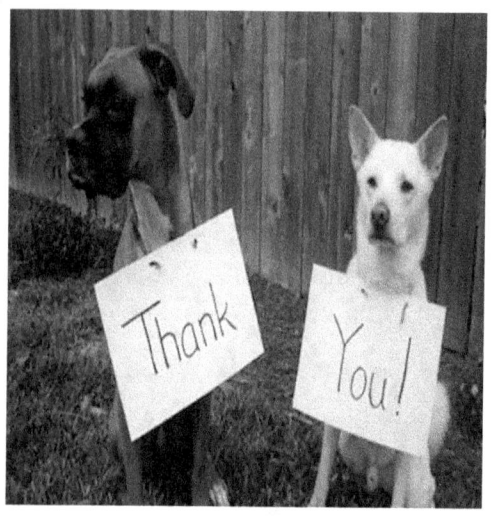

Finally, if you enjoyed this book, then I'd like to ask you for a favor, would you be kind enough to leave a review for this book on Amazon? It'd be greatly appreciated!

Thank you and good luck!

www.ingramcontent.com/pod-product-compliance
Lightning Source LLC
Chambersburg PA
CBHW062050280526
45788CB00003B/1173